REAL life GUIDES

THE BEAUTY INDUSTRY

TARA FALLON

3RD EDITION

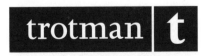

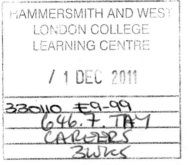
Real Life Guide to the Beauty Industry

This 3rd edition published in 2011 by Trotman, an imprint of
Crimson Publishing, Westminster House, Kew Road, Richmond,
Surrey TW9 2ND.

Author of this 3rd edition: Tara Fallon
Author of previous editions: Samantha Taylor

© Trotman Publishing 2007, 2011
1st edn published by Trotman & Co Ltd in 2004
© Trotman & Co Ltd 2004

ISBN: 978-1-84455-232-0

British Library Cataloguing in Publication Data
A catalogue record for this book is available from the British
Library

Typeset by IDSUK (DataConnection) Ltd
Printed and bound in the UK by Ashford Colour Press,
Gosport, Hants

THE BEAUTY INDUSTRY

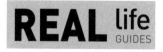
REAL life
GUIDES

Practical guides for practical people.

In this increasingly sophisticated world the need for manually skilled people to build our homes, cut our hair, fix our boilers, and make our cars go is greater than ever. As things progress, so the level of training and competence required of our skilled manual workers increases. In this series of career guides from Trotman, we look in detail at what it takes to train for, get into, and be successful at a wide spectrum of practical careers.

The Real Life Guides aim to inform and inspire young people and adults alike by providing comprehensive yet hard-hitting information about what it takes to succeed in these careers.

Other titles in this series are:

The Armed Forces

Business, Administration & Finance

Care, Welfare & Community Work

Carpentry & Cabinet Making

Catering

Childcare

Construction

Creative Industries

Electrician

Engineering Technician

Hairdressing

Hospitality & Events Management

Information & Communications Technology (ICT)

Manufacturing & Product Design

The Motor Industry

Plumbing

The Police Service

Retailing

Sport & Active Leisure

Travel & Tourism

Working Outdoors

Working with Animals & Wildlife

Working with Young People

CONTENTS

ABOUT THE AUTHOR

Tara Fallon worked for five years as a personal stylist (which included make-up application) before retraining and starting a new career as a careers adviser.

INTRODUCTION

Are you the kind of person who spends all their free time looking for the most up-to-date beauty news? Or trawling the internet looking for make-up tutorials? Well, why not make it pay?

The beauty industry is a fascinating and successful industry providing secure and interesting employment prospects. Many experienced therapists become successful business people, demonstrating a high level of skill and dedication, and there are even degrees available in beauty subjects, so you can still go to college, even university, if you eventually choose this option, to study something you love. Although traditionally considered a 'female' profession, the beauty industry is also fast opening up to men, who seem particularly drawn to make-up artistry and beauty consultancy, and some are now considering beauty therapy as a career.

> 66 The beauty industry is a fascinating and successful industry providing secure and interesting employment prospects. 99

If you are considering a career in the beauty industry, this book will provide you with the information you most need to make an informed decision about whether you should enter it.

In the Real Lives chapters in this book – Chapters 4, 6 and 9 – you'll find case studies which show what real beauty professionals are doing in their jobs and the advice they can offer you. But let's have a look at what's coming up in the other chapters of this book.

▶ **Chapter 1: Success story.** If you want to make a really successful career for yourself in beauty, read Chapter 1 for some great inspiration. Samantha Fane, who has carved out a fantastic career for herself, shares her story and offers tips on how to make your dream career a reality.

▶ **Chapter 2: What is the beauty industry?** In Chapter 2 we'll look at the beauty industry as a whole and some trends in products over the ages. This will give you a good grounding in the industry. This chapter also covers the different places that beauty professionals can find work, some of which may surprise you!

▶ **Chapter 3: What are the jobs?** There are an enormous range of jobs available and beauty professionals tend to be skilled in a number of them. In this chapter, we'll take a look at a range of roles in the industry; from entry level right up to more managerial or highly qualified positions.

▶ **Chapter 5: Tools of the trade.** In Chapter 5, we'll consider some of the most important skills you will need to be a beauty professional and whether you are the right kind of person to work in this industry. You should come away with the understanding that while the industry may be glamorous and creative, you also have to work hard and gain qualifications. Making people beautiful requires a lot of commitment, self-discipline and study; and you will also have to be the kind of person who gets on well with other people.

▶ **Chapter 7: FAQs.** This chapter will answer all the questions you need straight, honest answers to. How can I become a tattoo artist? Am I going to get lots of holidays?

Do I need to be beautiful to work in the industry? Have a look through this chapter so that you know exactly what to expect when you enter the industry.

▶ **Chapter 8: Qualifications and training.** Discover the most common qualifications in beauty subjects and try and make sense of what you should be studying now – and what you should be studying later, once you are in practice. Remember, all industries change, so never stand still: always be aware of how people buy beauty products and treatments and continually push your employer for as much training as you can get, particularly in new therapies and technologies.

▶ **Chapter 10: The last word.** By the time you reach this chapter you will have a really good idea about what working in the beauty industry involves. Try the light-hearted quiz in this chapter to see if you have what it takes to become a beauty professional!

This book will provide you with references to further information (see Chapter 11); but remember, if there's anything you're not sure about, discuss it with your school careers adviser, with Connexions or with careers advisers in your community. Two heads are better than one and these careers professionals will also help you to clarify your ideas about what kind of a person you are and whether you should choose the beauty industry as a future career.

CHAPTER 1
SUCCESS STORY

Vital Stats: Samantha Fane

Profession: Beauty clinic manager
First job: Representative for Avon cosmetics
Career high point: Managing her own salon aged 21

Samantha is the clinic manger of Renew Medica (one of 14 successful medical aesthetics clinics across London). She is responsible for managing three staff and providing a place for doctors and nurses to perform treatments like Botox, which removes facial lines. She has introduced lines of skincare and cosmetic products to the clinic which you can't buy on the high street, and she is also responsible for maintaining these stocks. She also has to decide the ambience (atmosphere) and interior decoration which is 'really interesting work as I have to decide what kind of setting my clients would find most relaxing and then organise for the clinic to be set up that way.'

Samantha began her career in 1992 when she took an International Health and Beauty Certificate (IHBC), and she developed good contacts on her course. Throughout her career most of her work has come from building good contacts from education and jobs.

Samantha's first job was as a representative for Avon, where some of her friends were also working. It was a useful first start, introducing Samantha to the idea of making sales and developing good product knowledge. She continued to offer beauty treatments to friends and family at the same time and she was able to develop this into a good business.

By the time she was 21 years old, Samantha was managing her own salon. 'I was quite young to be doing this kind of work, but my success was down to the contacts that I had built up – everyone had belief in my enthusiasm, my ability to work hard and my increasing industry knowledge and they felt these were the most important factors for choosing a manager.' Samantha's 1990s clinic was quite different from a clinic you would see today, offering toning-tables and tanning machines, now there are two rooms with couches for electrical procedures.

At this time, Samantha began to specialise in massage, including Shiatsu, and, after a long application process, she was lucky enough to be selected for Virgin Atlantic, offering massage and manicures on-board to first-class passengers. This job was both glamorous and demanding – 'we travelled to far-away places such as New York and Japan and China where relatively few Westerners had been, but it could be very tiring to give massages at 3a.m., when my body clock had not adapted – I needed to be professional at all times, no matter how I felt!'

After five and a half years, Samantha felt that the lack of routine in her working hours was no longer the right thing for her and she became a sales representative for an organisation called Hive of Beauty, selling waxing products and other beauty products throughout the south of England. This work was much more target-driven than the usual sales work carried out by beauty professionals, but Samantha said she had a real belief in her products and she was able to work successfully, always networking and making sure that every contact was pleased with her work and her personal skills. She went into another sales role with Gloprofessional after this, working with mineral make-up and aesthetic skincare for a year and a half.

> **❝** . . . everyone had belief in my enthusiasm, my ability to work hard and my increasing industry knowledge and they felt these were the most important factors for choosing a manager. **❞**

Again, through contacts Samantha made her most recent career move and became clinic manager for Renew Medica – they had been one of her top clients. She was able to bring a range of skills to this job, including considerable work experience as a beauty therapist, previous managerial experience and excellent sales and people-facing skills. Samantha points out that her job is not quite the same as a traditional beauty therapist because her work is 'more scientific: I have to learn more technology and keep up with rapid changes in technology. My work merges beauty and aesthetics and some customers feel it is more effective and offers quicker results than traditional beauty treatments.'

Samantha is very happy in her job. She loves to advise on products in which she has a genuine interest and she prefers a job in which she is working with people. Like other beauty professionals interviewed for this book, she feels rewarded by inspiring confidence in her clients and feels that some of her work can be life-changing – 'We had a lady with a lot of facial hair who lost a lot of self-esteem when only traditional treatments like electrolysis or threading were available – they just couldn't get rid of the hair. Laser removal actually worked, though, and this lady was able to face the world again.'

> 66 My work merges beauty and surgery and some customers feel it is more effective and offers quicker results than traditional beauty treatments. 99

Samantha does admit there are some negative sides to her job – she works quite unsociable hours, as she needs to be available to busy customers. She also feels that customers can be unrealistic about what they expect from the service and need to be continually reminded that some treatments (e.g. acne treatments) just need a while to work.

She needs to exercise a lot of patience and to keep smiling and be positive all the time – but this is all part of having excellent customer service skills; and indeed Samantha has managed to make personal friends of customers through having worked well with them over an extended period of time. She must also be on her feet for long periods of time, which she feels can be a disadvantage, but she wears support tights to help!

Despite being content with her job, Samantha remembers to continually retrain and think of the future. She is taking a management qualification offered by her employer – she's aware that you often need a qualification to match your experience. She has also, in the past, taught groups of 16- to 19-year-olds as part of their NVQ training ('rewarding', she says, 'but sometimes they don't concentrate enough!'). Either way, she has made it her business to have as many options available to her as possible, using the many skills she's developed over the years.

Samantha's top tip

66 The key to success in the beauty industry is to be always looking ahead and retraining. 99

CHAPTER 2
WHAT IS THE BEAUTY INDUSTRY?

BEAUTY THEN AND NOW

Beauty products: a brief history

Throughout history, both women and men have used beauty and cosmetic products to improve their personal appearance. We can see ancient pots of Egyptian eyeliner in museums and history tells us that Elizabethan women used lead-based make-up to whiten their skins – but, unfortunately, because lead is poisonous this caused terrible facial scarring and a number of illnesses such as gout.

It goes to show, however, that people have always been interested in improving their appearance and there have always been specialists available to help prepare and apply products and treatments.

Beauty fashions come and go, though. In the UK in Victorian times, using anything other than the most natural products, such as lavender water, was frowned upon, but beauty salons became more popular in the 20th

> ## ⚡ NEWSFLASH!
> Today the beauty industry is so big that beauty products are sold even in supermarkets and the British consumer spends over nine billion pounds every year.

century; and when Selfridges opened in London in 1909, it displayed cosmetics that women could buy openly for the first time.

Recent developments in the industry

There have in the last decade been a number of developments in the beauty industry which will continue to be popular for some time, so as an aspiring beauty practitioner you will need to know how to perform at least some of these treatments.

Holistic products

It's fashionable at the moment to seek alternative solutions to healthcare and beauty, and some very successful companies have been combining homoeopathy with beauty to provide treatments which take care of one's health as well as improving one's appearance, for example by using a 'holistic' approach – analysing stress levels, diet and emotional well-being – to sell both beauty and healthcare packages.

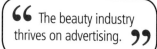

66 The beauty industry thrives on advertising. **99**

Some companies find it worthwhile to develop their own lines – or sell other manufacturers' products – which have been created from homoeopathic or 'natural' ingredients rather than stocking more traditional products. In an industry which thrives on advertising, many new products, including ingredients such as shea butter or jojoba oil, appear to be here to stay. For the same reason, tanning booths are used less, as public awareness of skin cancer continues to rise.

Check it out!
BABTAC: the British Association of Beauty Therapy and Cosmetology

Male beauty products

Men have been increasingly buying into beauty and some salons offer treatments, including waxing, fake tanning and manicures, that are specifically designed for men. There is even a new eyebrow bar in a

> **"** Good grooming is seen as necessary to workplace success. **"**

department store in London that caters solely for men – who are no longer ashamed to be seen publicly buying this service.

This is partly because good grooming is seen as necessary to workplace success and partly because women now expect men to spend more time on their appearance. Some cosmetics companies, such as Clinique, have developed skincare ranges targeting men and it has become much more common for male make-up artists to work in make-up promotion and sales, sometimes wearing full make-up as they do so. Women also increasingly buy beauty products for men.

The current state of the sector

The beauty industry is thriving and continues to be successful, despite the current recession. Cosmetics, for instance, are the easy sale in any designer range: most women find it easier to buy an Yves Saint Laurent lipstick than a dress. Most women and some men continue to prioritise care for their appearance, though they may now be buying from the high street rather than designer ranges and they will frequently see a new cosmetic or beauty product as an affordable, well-earned treat.

Beauty therapists report that their customers are still buying treatments, though there is a tendency to 'stretch' the time between treatments. Some treatments seem to be here to stay: Botox (an injectable liquid used to fill facial lines) has immediate, visible results and remains popular, despite the expense.

> ## ⚡ NEWSFLASH!
>
> Iman Cosmetics was founded in 1994 and was the first company to sell skincare and cosmetics to women with 'skin of colour'.

Antioxidants (natural ingredients which limit and repair damage to the skin's cells) also remain in demand and nail art remains very popular, as it is difficult to do this without professional help.

The future of the industry

The beauty industry will continue to provide good job opportunities, because people will always buy beauty products and treatments. However, to ensure you make your career a real success it is very important to always understand what your customers want and to understand what they buy and why.

Here are some predicted trends for the beauty industry.

- ▶ **Anti-ageing products.** Some beauty therapists have reported that they have seen an increase in anti-ageing products and treatments. This trend may continue as a bigger part of our population becomes older. Older clients also tend to have more disposable income as they earn more money and no longer support children.
- ▶ **Weight-loss programmes and nutrition.** Future beauty professionals may also find it useful to train in nutrition as rates of obesity continue to rise. Issues around obesity are continually reported in the media, so it is likely to lead to more people seeking treatment it they are overweight.
- ▶ **'Green' products.** We read about the environment in the media all the time now and a lot of people are very concerned about environmental issues. A limited range of organic beauty products have been available in health food

stores for several decades and June 2009 saw the first Fairtrade-certified beauty products available in the UK: these are 'green' and also ensure better working conditions for farmers in the Third World. Green practice will be

> 66 June 2009 saw the first Fairtrade-certified beauty products available in the UK. 99

extended into the actual running of beauty premises – for instance, computers will become more important as paper waste is cut – so keep practising your IT skills.

Here are some other treatments and products which may become more popular.

- ▶ **Gemstones**, which are supposed to have healing properties. Some cosmetics companies are already adding gemstones to face powders and lip glosses and there are a variety of beauty treatments available designed to boost your energy or relax you while at the same time improving your appearance.

- ▶ **Alternatives to cosmetic surgery.** Cheaper and easier alternatives such as injectable fillers and laser technology are becoming more popular, particularly as they offer quick and visible results which are important to clients with busy lives.

It's important to remember that consumers continually change the products they buy, so they will readily buy into change (change their choice of product), due to powerful advertising (such as make-up adverts on the television).

> ⚡ **NEWSFLASH!**
> The first ever nail polish was a mixture of sheep's fat and blood, used by the Romans!

11

WHERE WOULD YOU WORK?

The beauty industry extends to a wide variety of different settings, some of which involve moving from place to place as part of the job. Now that you have an idea of what the current state of the beauty sector is, read on to find out where you could find yourself working.

- ▶ **Salons** employ a variety of beauty professionals in order to provide as wide a range of services as possible – bigger organisations will be able to offer in-house training or fund new training. Some beauty therapists and nail technicians rent premises in a hairdressing salon.

- ▶ **Hotels.** Many beauty professionals are employed in these leisure premises, taking sales opportunities from their clients' sense of relaxation and well-being. You will not be required to build a regular clientele, but will be encouraged to market successfully to meet your salon's sales targets. Some larger hotels have spa areas that service local people as well as tourists.

- ▶ **Spas**, which offer a wider range of health, beauty and fitness services and employ professionals to cater for all these services. They differ from salons in that they have water facilities, such as saunas and pools, and offer treatments based around these in addition to more traditional salon-based treatments.

- ▶ **Health farms**, usually based in relaxing countryside settings. Clients visit these to get away from their daily worries and to go home feeling refreshed. Health farms will offer a very wide range of health and beauty treatments.

- ▶ **Care homes and hospitals** also require beauty therapists, masseuses and make-up artists to work a few hours of the week. They find it improves the self-esteem and morale of their patients and encourages the healing process. You might be expected to show that you already have experience with elderly or sick people and you should be aware that it's not always easy to work in settings like these – however, many people find the work very rewarding as they feel they are helping people who are particularly in need of it.

▶ **Airports** increasingly offer a range of therapy services, including manicures and massage – this is a good sales opportunity as travellers frequently have a number of hours to fill before check-in, and want to relax and feel more glamorous by the end of the journey. At a large international airport, you will have the opportunity to work with people from all over the world, so be prepared to work with people whose English might not be very good or who may have different cultural ideas about politeness.

▶ With experience, you may find employment on **cruise ships** or in **foreign holiday resorts**, where you will be expected to offer a variety of traditional and new treatments: the pay is above average for the industry, and contracts last an average of three to six months. You will also receive accommodation, food and travel costs. Beauty therapy is extremely popular in most countries and opportunities exist globally for qualified professionals, some travelling as far as the Middle East, Australia or South America.

> 66 With experience, you may find employment on cruise ships or in foreign holiday resorts. 99

BEAUTY INDUSTRY QUIZ ❓

Test yourself to see how much you know about this exciting industry!

1 What's the best reason to decide upon a career in the beauty industry?

A. I want a glamorous job with lots of travel

B. I love beauty: I can bring a genuine enthusiasm to my work and I'm prepared to work hard so I can develop my practice

C. It was the most convenient course for my timetable/locality

2 What do people want from modern beauty treatments?

A. Expensive products that feel nice

B. To spend hours relaxing

C. Quick, effective, visible results

3 Which of these hair removal treatments is most effective?

A. Threading

B. Electrolysis

C. Laser removal

4 How long has beauty been an industry?

A. Always

B. Since Victorian times

C. From the 20th century, when department stores began to openly stock beauty products

5 **Where would you expect to work as a beauty professional?**
A. Almost anywhere
B. Just in beauty salons
C. In places where people want to relax, like hotels and spas

6 **Is the beauty industry just for women?**
A. Yes: only women are interested in beauty
B. Not sure: men might be interested but they might not be able to get the work
C. No: men are already a thriving part of the beauty industry

7 **What are the most important treatments to learn as a beauty therapist?**
A. Manicures
B. Facials
C. The ones that sell best

ANSWERS

1 **B** – You'll need a real interest in your products, because you'll have to work with them all the time, and a real interest in the industry because that's where you'll spend all your working life.

2 **C** – The other answers can be true, but people lead very busy lives and on the whole want to pay for treatments that are quick and have very obvious results.

3 **C** – Laser removal is currently the most cutting-edge technology. It is worth learning these additional skills so you can charge more, and be more valuable to a potential employer.

4 **A** – References to beauty products have been found in the world's earliest records. Check your local museum and see what you can find!

5 **A** – A very wide variety of businesses can employ beauty professionals because so many customers want the services.

6 **C** – Check out YouTube for men's creative make-up tutorials, or go to the more adventurous beauty counters in your local department store.

7 **C** – Clients want different treatments all the time – you will always have to know what sells best.

Quick recap!

✓ You will have to keep up to date with all the latest developments in beauty treatments if you want to make your mark in this industry.

✓ To be really successful, you must understand what your customers want, and why.

✓ You can work in a huge variety of settings.

✓ There are lots of global opportunities for qualified professionals.

CHAPTER 3
WHAT ARE THE JOBS?

There are many different types of job available in the beauty industry. You can choose to work in one job that interests you most, or you can mix and match jobs to build a variety of knowledge that you can sell to employers. Most people in the industry will tend to do the latter, and some people will mix self-employment with working in paid jobs while they build up their business.

> ## ⚡ NEWSFLASH!
> Statistics show that, of all workers in the UK, beauty therapists and hairdressers are the happiest.

The way you work will be fairly similar across the range of jobs. With the exception of teachers, make-up artists and cosmetic scientists, beauty professionals generally work shifts, which will include evening and weekend work, in order to maximise sales. They will work between 37 and 40 hours a week, unless building their own business, working on a tight contract (such as a make-up artist working towards filming deadlines) or combining jobs.

Beauty professionals who work for themselves (freelance) can combine a

> ## TOP TIP! _i_
> You will need to make sure you are always aware of current treatments and new developments in beauty and you will need to regularly update your skills, so you must have a genuine interest in beauty.

number of temping jobs (taking on work for a period of a few weeks and months) with more permanent jobs, or with building up their own client base.

Information about new developments is easy to access once you are working in the industry, but you will also need to keep an eye on good-quality fashion/industry publications (see Chapter 11 for a list of ones to read).

WHAT KINDS OF JOBS ARE AVAILABLE?

Receptionist (beauty salon)

Receptionists are the customers' first point of contact with the beauty business, so they must ensure a friendly and attractive welcome. You will meet and greet clients, book appointments and deal with any queries or complaints that the customer might have, including organising the therapists' diaries and taking payments.

> **66** If you want to become a beauty therapist, you will have to take additional beauty qualifications. **99**

You will gain knowledge of a beauty therapist's role and treatment/ product knowledge, by observing how they work, and this could be a good starting point for a career in beauty. If you want to become a beauty therapist, you will have to take additional beauty qualifications.

Beauty therapist

There are a wide range of therapists available, all providing different services and using different products. If this is an area that interests you, you'll find that the following typical activities apply to all beauty therapy roles.

▶ You will use specialist knowledge to correctly work out any problems that your client may have (such as acne) and give correct treatment or advice.

▶ You will use professional tools and equipment (e.g. electrolysis equipment), which make treatments more effective. These require specialist training to ensure you can operate them safely.

▶ You must prove that you have a sound understanding of how to provide treatments safely and hygienically, according to health and safety standards.

▶ You will also keep a close watch on your clients' progress, perhaps through a number of visits, and change the treatments if necessary.

▶ You will also be expected to be able to find up-to-date information about new treatments and products and retrain where necessary.

Traditional beauty therapists administer treatments to clients to improve their personal appearance and also to relieve stress and improve their clients' sense of well-being and confidence. Treatments may include:

▶ facials to improve the appearance of the skin

▶ removing surplus hair by waxing, electrolysis and sugaring

▶ eyebrow shaping and threading

▶ eyelash colouring and the application of semi-permanent make-up

▶ spray tanning and UV tanning

▶ programmes designed to reduce cellulite (the lumpy texture sometimes found under the surface of the skin)

▶ non-surgical facelifts

▶ weight-loss programmes and body wraps (e.g. seaweed wraps) designed to help clients temporarily lose weight.

> 66 Some treatments, such as Botox, must be performed by medical professionals. 99

You will be expected to share reception duties, if necessary, booking appointments and greeting clients. You will maintain records of clients' treatment and product history and you will also be expected to sell products.

Some treatments, such as Botox, must be performed by medical professionals who have done additional training and have the correct medical insurance, but you will find yourself using a variety of different products, including chemical, organic and herbal, depending on what type of salon you work in – so beware of any skin allergies!

Check it out!
NASMAH: National Association of Screen Make-up Artists and Hairdressers

Some therapists choose to work for one particular well-known brand like Elemis or Dermalogica, in which case you will only be able to work with these products.

Complementary (holistic) therapist

Complementary (holistic) therapists work in the same way as more conventional beauty therapists, but they emphasise well-being and spirituality.

Treatments may include the following.

▶ **Massage therapy** to stimulate and improve the client's sense of well-being and/or improve the general appearance of the skin. There are many types of massage now available, the most famous being Thai and Swedish (using different hand techniques) and, though they are recognised as a medical discipline, it is not necessary to come from a medical background to perform them – most masseuses develop an interest through an interest in holistic well-being.

▶ **Infant massage** is also becoming popular – a therapist with a massage qualification can relax a baby (for example, causing it to cry less) and show the parent how to massage the child. The therapist may specialise in one type of massage or may be able to perform a number of different kinds.

▶ **Sports massage** is normally performed by a physiotherapist, but some massage therapists will also offer the service. The work may be performed either through the clothing or directly onto the skin and the therapist may use oils or creams. Massage therapists can work in a number of locations, including spas and salons, rented rooms in gyms and also in department stores selling products to customers. Agencies may also send them to workplaces and to events.

HOLISTIC THERAPIES

▶ **Aromatherapy:** preparing, mixing and applying oils to the client's skin in order to help with stress and treat skin problems. You will also record details of the client's medical history, diet and lifestyle so that you can decide the right essential oils to use.

▶ **Indian head massage:** massaging the scalp and hair to release negative energy, help with stress and encourage hair growth and condition.

▶ **Acupuncture:** inserting needles into specific acupuncture 'points' to help with both health and beauty problems. Practitioners say that acupuncture can cure a variety of beauty problems, including acne and other skin disorders, and that it can also help with weight loss.

▶ **Henna body art:** applying henna paste in intricate designs to the face or body. This practice originated in some Asian cultures and has become popular in the UK.

▶ **Reflexology** is based on the idea that 'reflex points' on the feet are connected to related areas throughout the body.

Reflexologists massage these points to release energy, which improves the appearance and health of the client. If they work in a spa, reflexologists often include soaking, wrapping, scrubbing, heating, towelling, aromatherapy or colour therapy as part of the treatment, so that the experience seems more luxurious.

There has been much argument recently about whether such treatments work, and holistic therapists voluntarily regulate themselves. This means that they have to perform to a certain quality and be of a certain standard to advertise their services. The Federation of Holistic Therapists, for example, requires members to follow a code of professional practice and offers training.

Medical aestheticians/electrotherapists

Medical aestheticians and electrotherapists work to achieve the same effect as beauty therapists. You will already have experience in traditional beauty therapy, but will need additional training. You will never practise surgery but you will use non-invasive (not cutting through the skin) surgery to provide more effective results than traditional treatments. Some examples of this are:

Check it out!
The Federation of Holistic Therapists: www.fht.org.uk.

▶ **ultratone:** stimulates the muscles electronically to alter and trim the body

▶ **laser hair removal:** using laser light to remove surplus facial or bodily hair

▶ **photo rejuvenation:** applying pulses of light to improve skin damage

▶ **micro-dermabrasion:** skin peeling to improve acne or skin pigmentation (blotches of colour)

▶ **complexion analysis system:** using skin mapping digital imaging technology. This technology assesses invisible

sun damage and skin condition and the therapist can
provide treatments to prevent the damage becoming worse.

As a medical aesthetician, you will
work in specialised clinics and must
be registered with the Healthcare
Commission as you will be using
potentially dangerous equipment.

> ⚡ **NEWSFLASH!**
> Some medical aestheticians
> have studied more anatomy
> and physiology than nurses!

If you work in a spa, you will be expected to provide an
additional range of services, including thalassotherapy (which
includes seaweed wraps and mud baths to cleanse skin and
reduce the appearance of cellulite) and Rasul (a steam and
mud treatment designed to improve the skin and prepare
the muscles for massage). A spa will normally offer in-house
training for this.

You will start in the industry by becoming a salon trainee
or assistant therapist. Salaries vary across the country and
according to age, but they start at around £15,000 and
may be topped up with commission and tips. You may also
be self-employed, going to clients' homes as required or
renting premises from another
business, in which case your
salary will depend on how
much you charge and how
much business you get.

> **Check it out!**
> BISA: British International Spa
> Association, www.spaassociation.
> org.uk.

A beauty therapist with around three years' experience and
a level 3 qualification may progress to senior therapist. You
will then be expected to supervise other staff and help with
their training.

With more experience, you might consider managing a beauty
premises for an employer or managing your own premises.

Beauty consultants

Beauty consultants advise on cosmetics, perfume and skincare products and sell them to the public. They demonstrate products, so they must be familiar with their range and some basic knowledge of skincare. If you became a beauty consultant, you would be responsible for displaying your products in an eye-catching manner and would have to re-order when necessary.

Beauty retail has the third largest sales turnover in retail – so this is a busy work environment.

Beauty consultants work in department stores, brand stores (e.g. Shu Uemura or MAC, which both have small retail premises and employ trained make-up artists) or independently, buying stock and selling it to their own customers, for example by working for Avon.

⚡ NEWSFLASH!
UK consumers spend £5 billion every year on cosmetics.

If you are a fairly confident person and already have knowledge of other products, this might be a good way to start gaining work experience, fitting it in while you're at college.

Some companies, like Clinique, recruit and provide in-house training but beauty consultants are generally employed by agencies on a casual basis and work for a base rate and commission (they earn money depending on how much they sell) – this means it's important that they make sales. Salaries are generally commission-based, so if you were working on a retail premises, you would receive a basic wage of

around £6 per hour (although this will depend on your age).
You could also receive discounted cosmetics as you will be
expected to wear the company's own range. You might be
employed at airports to sell duty-free products.

As a beauty consultant you can progress in your career
to manage other staff and eventually become a beauty
accounts manager. You will then be responsible for increasing
sales at your counter, inventing ways of encouraging more
custom, promoting your employer's brand, and training and
motivating new staff. This is a highly sales-driven job but no
specific qualifications are required – only sales performance
and knowledge of the products. Beauty accounts managers
can earn between £16,000 and £40,000 p.a., depending on
success and experience.

Make-up artists

Make-up artists are never employed on a full-time basis, but
they can develop their business in a variety of ways.

▶ Working with an image stylist to provide a thorough
   restyling service, or helping customers with their make-up
   for special one-off occasions such as weddings.

▶ Working on fashion shows or editorial shoots to improve
   the appearance of the model.

▶ Working in TV/film with other fashion or media
   professionals for a variety of purposes, including:

   o improving the appearance of TV personnel so they
      appear to best effect in front of camera

   o creating special effects, such as ageing the actor or
      creating the effect of wounds/burns/bruising.

▶ Some make-up artists work with clients to apply specialised
   brands of skin make-up (e.g. Dermablend) to cover severe

skin defects. These products are quite different from high street make-up and their application can create a drastic improvement in quality of life for people with scars, burns or acne.

As a make-up artist you will gain much of your work through networking (making the right kind of contacts), so you would need to think flexibly about the way you work. You would work by contract, for as long as you were needed on a particular production, and this could include long hours and periods of time spent away from home.

▶ You need good product knowledge and must be able to work creatively, thinking 'outside the box' with your materials.

▶ You also need some understanding of basic hair styling (not cutting), e.g. using curling tongs and applying wigs and need to know how to use specialised products like false hair, theatre grease and prosthetics.

▶ You would have to research some of your material, to provide the most accurate designs and be aware of current trends in design to best interpret producers' ideas.

▶ Courses are available that teach important skills; however, experience and contacts in the fashion and beauty industries are more important than qualifications.

66 Make-up artists may also be paid to promote make-up products and will certainly receive a lot of free make-up! 99

Salaries vary, depending on how much and what type of work you can find, though the Broadcasting, Entertainment, Cinematograph and Theatre Union (BECTU) can advise on rates of pay: a make-up artist currently earns around £200–£250 before tax for a 10-hour day, depending on employer. A make-up artist who can build up a popular reputation through vlogs/blogs (these are website pages often dedicated to the subject – vlogs are videoed) may also be paid to promote make-up products and will certainly receive a lot of free make-up!

Image consultants

Image consultants have become increasingly popular in recent years following the success of TV programmes like Gok Wan's *How to Look Good Naked* and *Gok's Fashion Fix*. Like make-up artists, they work by building up their own businesses, relying on networking with other fashion or beauty professionals and building a good reputation among customers to encourage repeat business.

▶ Image consultants take responsibility for all their own marketing in fashion and retail publicity and work with clients to build up an idea of their lifestyle, manage their wardrobe, create a new style or refine an existing style.

▶ If you want to become an image consultant you must be able to identify different types of body shape and understand how fabric and colour can work to improve these shapes.

▶ Image consultants might work on one-off events, such as weddings or other special occasions, but sometimes they become trusted advisers, working with clients over a long period of time.

▶ This is not an entry-level job. Image consultants generally have to have years of experience in fashion or beauty before advertising as a professional image consultant, but some find it useful to take specialist courses available at some higher education institutions or through training from organisations such as Colour Me Beautiful, which may also employ image consultants on a self-employed basis. Image consultants who work for businesses may be employed to give talks or presentations to company staff for a variety of reasons, including raising morale, or may even be involved in restyling company uniforms.

▶ Some image consultants work in the media, preparing clients for interview, and some include articles in the national or local press as part of their portfolio (a CV of achievements).

▶ If you want to be an image consultant you will need a space in an office, shop or even your own home, in which clients can visit you, though you may find it useful to visit clients to view their wardrobe and gain a clearer understanding of their lifestyle. You may find it useful to invest in resources such as a mannequin, mirrors or natural lighting.

▶ Your hours would be flexible, based around the needs of your clients, and you would expect to work evenings and weekends. It is not possible to say what a starting salary is as this will be determined by the amount of work you find for yourself and the rates you charge (you should work this out by researching what your competition charges), but an experienced stylist who has built up a good reputation will expect to exceed £40,000 p.a.

> ## ⚡ NEWSFLASH!
> The beauty industry in China is booming – over 51% of salons opened in the past five years – so if you want to travel, China might be a good place to set up a business.

Nail technicians

Nail technicians usually work in nail studios, salons and stalls in department stores. A nail technician might work in clients' homes, rent a space in an existing beauty salon or hairdresser's work from home or work within another business such as a hotel, gym, department store or spa.

They perform basic manicures and pedicures and also apply artificial nails, acrylic extensions and decorations using coloured varnish, transfers, gems and glitter. They also sometimes use airbrushing techniques.

Nail technicians must check nails for disease and normally give a basic hand massage. With experience, some nail technicians will work with fashion designers and photographers for fashion shoots/photo shoots and many technicians will develop their own business. Salaries start at around £10,000 p.a.

Tattoo artists

Tattoo artists apply permanent artwork to their clients' skin using ink and electronically operated needles. They work independently, which means that they are responsible for building their own business. To start out as a tattoo artist you need to train as an apprentice for two to three years. You will also have to buy start-up equipment, which would cost about £4,000–£5,000. There are currently no courses you can do apart from an Apprenticeship (you will have to persuade a tattoo artist to take you on), and your studio must be registered with the local Environmental Health Department so that your work is regulated according to safety standards.

Your Apprenticeship will include not only learning to apply a tattoo accurately (many months' training in itself), but also how to use your tattoo machinery, health and safety and how to protect yourself and your clients from disease. Salaries range from £11,000 to £30,000, depending on experience and reputation. Remember that you will receive no government funding to do your training, so you must support yourself with another job at the same time. To find out what real life is like as a tattoo artist, turn to Chapter 9 to read about Dave O'Sullivan.

Cosmetic scientists

Cosmetic scientists work to develop new beauty products such as skincare, perfumes and make-up. They come from a scientific background but have an interest in beauty products and should be aware of what is already on the market and how the public have reacted to it, particularly if they are involved in research or product development.

> ⚡ **NEWSFLASH!**
>
> Chinese women used to blacken all their teeth – white teeth were considered very ugly.

They also get involved in designing packaging, making sure that the new products are safe and adhere to legal requirements, or testing raw ingredients to make sure they are safe and suitable. Much of this work will be performed in laboratories. It is possible to leave school after level 3 and become a laboratory assistant, building up further training on the job, but a degree in cosmetic science would be useful for this career. Therefore it is not an entry-level job for when you leave school. Salaries begin at around £18,000 p.a. and, with more experience, you might earn up to £50,000 p.a.

Teachers

Once you have gained industry experience, you might consider teaching. This is likely to take place in further and adult education colleges, though if you teach salon management you could also work in higher education. You will not need a degree but you will have to gain an additional teaching qualification. In addition to your knowledge of beauty therapy, you will have to plan lessons and to show the ability to manage a group of students, dealing with both professional and personal problems as they arise.

Depending where you work, you may also be target-driven – paid a bonus to keep students on the course and progress them into qualification. Salaries begin at around £22,000.

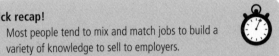

Quick recap!

✓ Most people tend to mix and match jobs to build a variety of knowledge to sell to employers.

✓ You should read lots of different good-quality beauty and fashion publications.

✓ To work in beauty you should have very good awareness of health and safety.

CHAPTER 4
REAL LIVES 1

LOURISHA WOODALL: BEAUTY THERAPIST

Lourisha is 20 years old and has been working in the beauty industry for about a year.

When she was at school, Lourisha didn't complete her GCSEs but was already very interested in beauty therapy. She contacted her local college in Birmingham and was invited in for an assessment in maths and English, which she passed at level 2. This meant that she could enrol on a level 2 NVQ in Beauty Therapy, which she completed over the next two years.

Lourisha enjoyed her course but found it 'harder than I expected: I was assessed in the college salon on a number of "cases" (beauty consultations) and I could only progress if I got each case right – it could be frustrating but it was important I learned everything thoroughly.'

She also had to learn about diet, exercise, sleep and other science-related subjects, such as how muscles, glands and blood work. She was fortunate enough to gain solid salon experience for five months and was one of the 50% who passed her course – despite 'the awful time when I first did electrolysis and accidentally burned a client's face!'

Lourisha wasn't able to find work as a beauty therapist immediately after leaving college, as the employers she approached felt she hadn't gained quite enough experience. Her first job was working as a receptionist in an office and, though she was a bit disappointed, Lourisha feels that this suited her at the time, because she was able to use her excellent customer service skills in this role. However, she did miss beauty and when her friends told her about a local nightclub's night vacancy for head masseuse in a 'chill room' she quickly applied. She had to offer head massages to clients who needed a little rest after all their dancing! 'This was a really fantastic job,' she says. 'You don't really think about working in a nightclub when you're studying but it's a very sociable way to earn a living – and NO, I wasn't allowed to drink!' Lourisha earned £16 for every 10- to 15-minute massage she gave (minus the club's rental, which was about £5).

> 66 I really feel I'm doing something useful for people – I can see the stress disappearing as I work. 99

Lourisha left Birmingham and moved to London after about a year. Despite the recession, she very quickly received two job offers, both of which she decided to accept. The first job offer was more nightclub work, though she is at a disadvantage in London because she doesn't drive and can't easily move from place to place. Her agency sends her not only to nightclubs, but to offices and events and exhibitions, where she massages clients sitting down in chairs; manipulating their heads and shoulders without oils to first relax and then energise the client.

The second job offer was a trainee spa therapist role. In addition to her £7 per hour salary (plus tips and commission), she has also received free on-the-job training to top up what she learned at college. This has included hot stone therapy and Shiatsu and Thai massage, which has given Lourisha a little more direction: she now feels that she would like to specialise in massage, especially Thai massage, because 'I really feel I'm doing something useful for people – I can see the stress disappearing as I work.'

She is also asking for any training she can receive in the more 'scientific' therapies, as she feels these are becoming increasingly popular and could provide additional income in the future.

As with all jobs, there is a downside: Lourisha is given additional time for consultation (asking the client health-related questions), post-consultation (arranging for the client to come back) and tidying the room and linen, but the work can be repetitive and monotonous and Lourisha is standing on her feet for long periods of time.

> 66 Making other people happy and improving their confidence is the most important thing for me. 99

However, despite this and despite the long hours that she is currently working, she describes herself as very happy – when asked what is the most important priority for her, she replied that 'making other people happy and improving their confidence is the most important thing for me'. A big part of all these jobs has been to make product sales, and Lourisha feels that she has been successful at this, mostly because 'if you build a good relationship with the customer, they get to know you and feel they can trust your advice'. Lourisha has enjoyed the sales side and feels she is good at meeting targets and making profit.

She would eventually like to own and manage her own salon premises but understands the importance of starting small. She has enrolled on an adult education course in marketing (she will cut down some of her agency hours to allow for this) as she has already begun to think about business opportunities to sell massage through GP referrals and in local care homes. 'I'm quite creative,' she says, 'and I would be able to produce all my own flyers and marketing literature and take them around to interested businesses.'

> 66 If you build a good relationship with the customer, they get to know you and feel they can trust your advice. 99

Lourisha has no regrets about choosing beauty as her profession, despite difficulties in gaining employment at first and worries about having to co-ordinate a number of part-time roles. She feels that the more experience she gets, the more focus she gets and she is very positive and has lots of ideas about her future.

CHAPTER 5
TOOLS OF THE TRADE

When you are deciding the kind of job you want to do, one of the things you have to think about is why you want to do it.

You might decide you want to work in a salon or spa because it's a very relaxed environment, or you might want to work on a cruise ship because it's exciting to travel. Perhaps you want to be a make-up artist because you will meet celebrities; or you might want to be a plastic surgeon because you'll make lots of money. If these values are important to you, that's fine, but you need to look at the bigger picture – you should also consider whether the beauty industry matches your skills and personal qualities.

IS THE BEAUTY INDUSTRY RIGHT FOR YOU?

The beauty industry requires skilled workers and potential employers will expect to see evidence that you are very enthusiastic and have

66 As you progress in your career, you will be expected to show considerable knowledge of what products are available and how they work. 99

well-thought-out reasons for wanting to do your chosen job. Be clear about why you want to work in this industry and what you can contribute to it.

Product knowledge

It would make sense that, before you begin your beauty career, you should already have an interest in beauty or make-up products and their application – you don't have to actually know about everything on the market, but if you're the kind of person who regularly reads the 'beauty' sections of magazines or information on the internet, or who spends a lot of time doing your own or your friends' make-up, simply because you enjoy it, that's a good start. As you progress in your career, you will be expected to show considerable knowledge of what products are available and how they work.

Professional appearance

Remember that potential employers and customers will expect their very first impression of you to reflect the services you offer – you must be well groomed and made up! You must also avoid smelling of anything strong, such as garlic or cigarette smoke, as these may be off-putting to other people and will potentially lose business for your company. You will be expected to wear a salon uniform, even when training, and you must keep your hair, nails and make-up neat and tidy.

TOP TIP! *i*

You should avoid smelling of anything strong, such as garlic or cigarette smoke, as these may be off-putting to other people.

Creativity

You may need a certain amount of creativity, though this depends on the job. A make-up artist will often be expected to be highly creative: they will be the pioneers of the catwalk or fashion editorial; and their designs often create other fashion movements.

If you are a make-up artist working as a beauty consultant (and this will happen with brands like MAC and Illamasqua), you may be expected to sell your products as creative ones, in which case you might be expected to help customers to make flamboyant designs with their make-up. As a make-up artist you will also be given a brief (information about the desired result) and will be expected to use your own ideas to come up with results.

You may also be expected to show a certain amount of creativity as an image consultant: this depends on your client and the brief they give you – for example, working on a small budget to redesign someone's wardrobe, or designing a uniform which will keep all staff happy may require more imagination than working towards a specific event like a wedding, where a certain amount of style 'rules' must be followed.

> 66 To work in beauty, you must be the type of person who can finish a job well. 99

Attention to detail

Successful creativity is partially about attention to detail. To work in beauty, you must be the type of person who can finish a job well. Faults in make-up application will show on camera, faults in waxing technique will be obvious to the customer and a product sold with the addition of appealing packaging will encourage further spending. A nail technician is expected to make flawless, intricate designs – you can't be the kind of person who will leave glue showing or paint out of line.

Perception

Attention to detail is very much about observation. This level of observation is called 'perception' and it will allow you to pick up on clients' body language and tone of voice: the basis of good customer service.

Customer service

The most important of your 'soft' skills is your ability to relate well to your clients, and this is important in all the beauty industry jobs mentioned in this book. It will be part of your job to encourage repeat business and to make sales: most people buy into the beauty industry not only because they want to look good, but because they regard it as a leisure event ('me time'). Many of the skills listed below are part of good customer service skills.

Friendliness

It will be much easier for you to do your job if your customer feels that you are a friendly person who is genuinely interested in them and their problems. In addition to being confident and chatty with your clients, prepare to be sensitive to their needs: a massage therapist, for instance, may have to decide when to chat and when to be silent (your client might not always want to talk) – sometimes you will have

> **66** A customer will be more likely to trust your advice and feel comfortable . . . if they have built up a friendly relationship with you. **99**

to feel your way. A customer will be more likely to trust your advice and feel comfortable enough to buy into your services again if they have built up a friendly relationship with you.

Communication skills

These are an important part of customer service, team working and gaining employment. One of the most important things a potential employer will look for is your ability to meet them in the eye, smile and look confident. They will need to know that you can work well with other staff members and can take direction well. Equally, customers don't want to have to ask you to repeat yourself because you're mumbling or because they can't understand you, so speaking clearly in standard English is important.

Listening

Good listening skills are harder than you think! You must listen accurately and patiently to your customer. If you have a full diary, you may feel stressed about completing your customer's appointment on time: the temptation will be not to listen properly, but assume you know what they want, in which case you may not be giving a service that the customer wants. Make sure you can give your customer enough time to explain their problem accurately.

TOP TIP! *i*

One of the most important things a potential employer will look for is your ability to meet them in the eye, smile and look confident.

Maintaining boundaries

It is extremely important that you build a good relationship with your customer, but this relationship will change very quickly if the customer decides they didn't get the service they paid for. It is important that the customer remains aware that you are a friendly professional; otherwise they will take the sort of advantage that friends take.

Managing clients' expectations

Clients with less knowledge than you may very well expect that a massage will heal a back problem or an anti-wrinkle cream will permanently delete wrinkles. Beauty/massage therapists or nail technicians should be prepared for the times when they have to deal with confrontational customers who are frustrated by a lack of results – and this requires excellent customer service skills and the ability to remain calm, friendly and in control of the situation.

Honesty

You might sometimes have to balance professional honesty against the pressure to meet your sales target. Most therapists say that building up trust sells more products in the long run.

Sensitivity

You will also need to behave professionally around personal hygiene issues, such as clients who have not washed correctly before massage or who have a fungus on their nail when they want a pedicure. You will need to be sensitive enough not to embarrass your client but you will have to deal with the problem for health and safety reasons. Also, if you have enough sensitivity to deal nicely with the client, they are much more likely to return and use your services again.

> 66 Most therapists say that building up trust sells more products in the long run. 99

Sharing information

You will need to be able to explain clearly to the customer what you're doing and what products you're using so that they can make informed decisions.

Networking (making contacts)

People who are good at customer service tend to be good at networking, because they have developed the knack of making themselves likeable and, in some beauty industry jobs such as make-up artist, image consultant and beauty journalist, you will have to network hard to get work. You will have to start by building a portfolio (a 'catalogue' showing your work and listing clients or events) in these last three jobs and you might start networking by asking other fashion professionals to help you, on the basis that you all need free publicity – you might need a model to display your image consultancy skills, or a fashion designer to lend you some clothes, or a photographer who can display your work to the best advantage. You will need exactly the same approachable manner and good communication skills to sell your ideas to these professionals that you would need to build a good relationship with customers.

WORKPLACE SKILLS

Even in times of high unemployment in the UK, many employers have a hard time recruiting to fill their vacancies. The reason for this is that many candidates who are otherwise well qualified lack enough relevant workplace experience or have poorly developed workplace skills (for example, they might not be good at team working or communication skills or have much knowledge of how the workplace operates).

Most qualifications that will take you into the beauty industry will have to meet National

> **⚡ NEWSFLASH!**
>
> The record for the world's longest nails is held by Lee Redmond from the USA who grew them to 24 feet, 7.8 inches. Soaking them in olive oil helped the process.

Occupational Standards – these are established with employers who have already identified 'skills gaps' and this kind of skills development should be part of your course.

This is important to you because it is preparing you for the world of work and future employers will be very interested in these skills. Try to identify how this is happening – you should be able to know when you are working successfully as part of a team (for instance if you are completing a project with other students or if you have had to take responsibility for organising a project), because you will have to explain this when writing a CV or at interview.

Literacy/numeracy/IT

Keep in mind that employers also complain about candidates' poor literacy and numeracy – you need these skills nowadays in any industry, so make sure they are up to at least level 2 standard (more if you want to take a degree), even if they need lots of practice. You will also need IT skills – your duties will include stocktaking, re-ordering stock and perhaps using a database such as Premier Spa for booking clients.

> 66 You can't just ask people to help you if you're not willing to help yourself. 99

Punctuality and reliability

How you manage the workplace is something that comes with experience, so try to choose a course with a lot of work placements. A record of attending punctually, lasting a course or job without taking lots of sick leave, and also keeping your manager or tutor informed if there's a problem, is prized by future employers.

Never giving up

There will be problems, but if you give up because it all seems too difficult, you won't be a good beauty professional. As a beauty therapy apprentice from Lewisham College put it, 'you can't just ask people to help you if you're not willing to help yourself'.

Team working

Team working is a workplace skill that you will be definitely asked about – it is a favourite question of employers or colleges at interview. Team working is the ability to share information accurately and to work well with other professionals to create a supportive and successful work environment. Whether you are at college or already in the workplace, think about how you already do this on a daily basis – you might be working on a project with another student or you might be sharing ideas to come up with a solution to a problem.

⚡ **NEWSFLASH!**

Botox is made from botulinum toxin, the most poisonous substance known to man.

Business skills

Business skills is a known skills shortage in the beauty industry. The beauty industry continues to do well in recessions, though there is evidence that customers will buy from a lower price range. If you work as a beauty consultant on the Crème de la Mer counter, for example, you might find it harder to sell a £100 moisturiser, but Crème de la Mer will still expect to make its profits! You may have to deal with your own accounts and taxes, which means you will have to keep all your invoices/receipts; and good numeracy and remembering to meet tax deadlines will be essential.

Marketing skills

A beauty consultant may find it useful, and a beauty accounts manager will find it necessary, to show good marketing skills, working creatively to encourage customers to come to the counter. You will have to find out their contact details for further marketing and you must work imaginatively to keep customers interested enough to come back to your counter.

Creating a relaxed atmosphere

Therapists may be responsible for creating the ambience (atmosphere) of their salon to encourage custom and should at least understand how ambience is created.

Managerial skills

If you run your own salon, you will have to manage staff, which means you will need to understand employment law and recruitment. Managerial skills are different from being friendly and popular – you will have to find the right balance between being approachable enough for staff to feel comfortable about communicating problems but firm enough to maintain discipline. It's not easy – managerial skills are a very specific set of skills based on experience, so it's important that you gain lots of workplace experience before you consider setting up your own salon.

> ### ⚡ NEWSFLASH!
> Otzi the Iceman (excavated in the Alps in 1991) died 53 centuries ago. He had a total of 57 tattoos, which suggests that tattooing is one of our oldest beauty traditions.

If you are self-employed and working on your own, the chief skills you will need are reliability (a must for establishing a regular and satisfied clientele), good customer service and organisation, as you will be regularly doing lots of different jobs and keeping ahead of your stock requirements.

Positive attitude

A lot of job adverts for beauty professionals will ask for a positive attitude, and your school or college will also expect it. When you are out working, you will be part of a business which will want to grow and may face problems and challenges on the way – your employer will want to feel that they can rely on you to remain a cheerful member of the team and can continue to contribute by coming up with new ideas. You will also face problems with your coursework. No matter how interesting you find the subject, there are always going to be those moments when you just can't get a nail design right or you just can't

> 66 Your employer will want to feel that they can rely on you to remain a cheerful member of the team. 99

seem to work your electrolysis tools – but you have to remain positive and keep trying. All the case studies in this book emphasise the importance of never giving up!

Health and safety

An awareness of health and safety will be standard across the beauty industry, from cleaning rooms and linen between beauty treatments to keeping your make-up brushes sterilised between clients, to identifying skin or nail disease. You may be using potentially dangerous equipment or chemicals so you must be aware of how to use them safely.

Confidentiality

Your customers will also expect that everything they say to you, or any beauty issues which might arise, will remain confidential. In other words, you mustn't gossip – and you will probably sign a contract to agree to this when you start work.

Physical fitness

With the exception of nail technicians, professionals in the beauty industry generally work standing up for long periods of time and there may be only limited time for breaks, so you need lots of stamina. You will need to maintain a positive, upbeat attitude with all your customers even when you are tired or your feet are hurting, and this will be particularly important if you are working in a care home or hospital setting.

> 66 Your customers will also expect that everything they say to you, or any beauty issues which might arise, will remain confidential. 99

Quick recap!

✓ Be clear about why you want to work in this industry and what you can contribute.

✓ You need to be very perceptive to work in beauty. Reading your clients' body language is an important skill.

✓ Your client should trust you. Make sure you come across as friendly, open and honest.

CHAPTER 6
REAL LIVES 2

KATIE WILSON: BEAUTY ACCOUNTS MANAGER

Katie Wilson is a beauty accounts manager working in Harvey Nichols in London. She manages four top-of-the-range perfume brands (Creed, Etro, Caron and Robert Piguet) and comes from a beauty consultancy background.

'When I left school, I didn't really have very clear career plans. I'd always been really interested in skincare and perfumes and my mum had the great idea of approaching an agency who employed beauty consultants.'

The agency sent Katie out to work on make-up counters in department stores throughout London, including Harrods and Harvey Nichols, and Katie worked on various counters including Clinique and Estée Lauder. 'It was quite hard work; I had to make sure I looked really smart all the time and we always had to wear high heels – my feet were aching by the end of the day, but it did feel nice having to dress up.'

> 66 I was really good at marketing! I suppose, because I liked the products so much, I could see good ways of selling them. 99

Katie also began to develop different skills once she was working: 'I had no idea before I started this job, but I was really good at marketing! I suppose, because I liked the products so much, I could see good ways of selling them.' Katie also has very good people skills and encouraged customers to leave their contact details with her – she would then phone them, using incentives like discounts and launches of new products, to get them to return to the counter and buy more products. This proved to be very successful and Katie managed to increase sales so much that after two years she was promoted to account manager and supervisor for a fragrance company retailing at Harvey Nichols.

'It was quite a responsibility but I felt very proud that people were so impressed by my sales skills – these are definitely one of the most important skills you can have working on beauty counters.'

> ❝ Sales skills are definitely some of the most important skills you can have working on beauty counters. ❞

Katie was now managing four perfume brands: Caron, Creed, Etro and Robert Piguet – these brands are very prestigious, but because they are not advertised as much as well-known brands, they can be more difficult to sell, which can make Katie's job harder.

> ❝ A lot of people like to get this kind of work because they think it's nice to work with beauty products, and they don't necessarily realise that it can be a bit pressurised. ❞

Katie's job was now very different: 'I still sold products to customers sometimes, but really my job was about managing staff and considering long-term sales. We take on a lot of agency and promotional staff and, if they're a bit inexperienced, I have to work with them to make sure they know about the perfumes and also that they know there are sales targets involved – a lot of people like to get this kind of work because they think it's nice to work with beauty products, and they don't necessarily realise that it can be a bit pressurised.'

Katie also has to keep her staff motivated because sometimes they can be anxious if they are not making sales. 'If you want to make sales,' Katie says, 'you have to remain very enthusiastic and cheerful: customers really pick up on this and they will feel more interested in the products you're selling.'

Katie still uses her creative skills, always thinking about what she can do next to encourage customers to buy – this can be as simple as reorganising her counter or arranging information in a more eye-catching way, for instance by adding prices and essential information near till points.

> 66 If you want to make sales you have to remain very enthusiastic and cheerful: customers really pick up on this and they will feel more interested in the products you're selling. 99

She also still uses her customer service skills, talking on a regular basis with area managers and the buying office (and occasionally the European area manager).

She has to help them solve problems relating to stock, so she needs to be very confident and to communicate her ideas very clearly. She also has to do a lot of administration, putting together sales reports for management and also managing stock levels – so she has to have good literacy and numeracy skills.

> 66 I've really surprised myself – I feel I've built up a really successful career based on taking a fun job selling make-up. 99

Katie feels she is not particularly good with computers, but has recently completed a computer course because she does need IT skills to write up her reports.

She thinks the worst part of her job is 'the long hours and the fact I have to work really hard, but I think it's worth it because I get a bonus and a real sense of achievement'.

The best part is 'the fact that I've really surprised myself – I had no idea when I was at school that I was going to be good at marketing and sales. I feel I've built up a really successful career based on taking a fun job selling make-up.'

Katie's top tip

66 Be confident – try anything that comes your way because you don't know what you're good at until you try it! 99

CHAPTER 7
FAQs

You should already have gained a lot of information from reading the other chapters of this book. In this chapter we'll cover a range of questions that commonly arise.

Q 66 **What is the best qualification I can take if I want to be a beauty therapist?** 99

A In terms of employment, it doesn't really matter what the qualification is called, although you should do as high a level as you can. You would currently need at least a level 2 qualification to realistically find employment afterwards, but because competition is strong, it would be better if you could get a level 3 qualification.

Prioritise any course which can guarantee work experience and as much of it as possible. In terms of successfully studying, you should try and work out what would best suit you – some courses might have more written content than others, for instance.

Q 66 **I'm already studying a beauty qualification. What else can I do to improve my chances of getting work afterwards?** 99

A Consider getting a Saturday job. Even if it's just helping clean the salon, it means you're meeting people who may know of vacancies, who may put in a word for you if they are impressed with your attitude and who may even be in a position to employ you as a therapist once you've qualified.

 66 Where is the best place to study a beauty therapy NVQ level 2? 99

 The only way to find out is to attend the open days offered by further education colleges, and be prepared to ask questions. You should ask them if they can offer a work placement as part of their training package and how many hours it will involve – there should be a high content of workplace experience, not only because this is the way an NVQ is assessed but because it will give you the edge with future employers.

> **⚡ NEWSFLASH!**
>
> Cosmetics companies can grow sheets of human skin to test skin creams!

Be aware that if you start a course and have to withdraw because the college has failed to deliver the work placement, this may affect future funding for your education. Ask to see in-house salons and ask to speak to current students. Some colleges not only help you find work placements, but are on government targets to get students into employment, so ask about their links with employers and ask what kind of help you can get from the college in looking for work. Also ask what percentage of students successfully complete the course: if they give a low percentage, you should look for another college, even if they seem to be giving convincing reasons. Don't be afraid to ask them as many questions as you want: if you look like you want the best for yourself and your future, people will respect this.

> **66** Some colleges not only help you find work placements, but are on government targets to get students into employment. **99**

 66 I started my beauty therapy course, but the college has now told me I must find my own work placement. How should I go about this? 99

Enthusiasm and good presentation are most important in this situation. Prepare your CV and go into salons so that the manager can see you – in this industry, this approach is more effective than making phone calls asking for work placements. Use your communication skills to explain your situation clearly and make sure you know exactly how many hours to ask for and what your learning objectives are. Make sure you look happy, friendly and approachable. Be prepared to answer any questions on future career plans and why you're studying your current qualification. You might have to go to a number of different premises before you're successful, so it's important to remain optimistic.

> **TOP TIP!**
>
> To get a work placement, you might have to go a number of different premises before you're successful, so it's important to remain optimistic.

Q 66 I'm just about to finish my NVQ level 2. How do I find out about vacancies for in-flight beauty therapists? 99

A Airlines are currently cutting back on staff – it would be better to spend the next couple of years gaining some experience in a salon setting and then reconsidering your options. You would need to gain several years' experience before considering these jobs, anyway. If you currently have some experience, you may want to consider jobs on cruise ships – check Google for vacancies.

Q 66 I just want to be a self-employed therapist when I finish my NVQ – I don't want to work for an employer. Is this a good idea? 99

A If you already have experience of self-employment it might work. However, you will miss sharing practice with your colleagues, so your industry knowledge and techniques may not progress as much as they would if you worked on a beauty premises. If you don't have previous knowledge of self-employment, this will be the first time you have dealt with business matters. Have you considered how you will drum up business? How you will pay your bills if you can't get enough work? What it will be like dealing with all

TOP TIP!

Prioritise any course that can guarantee work experience and as much of it as possible.

your business problems on your own? It would be best to get some experience first: you can learn all these things from an employer and the knowledge will give you a better start. Also ask yourself why you don't want to work for an employer – if you haven't got enough people skills to take instructions from your manager or handle the rough and tumble of workplace life, you'll find it difficult to manage your customers – and that's really important if you're running your own business.

Q 66 I really want to be a nail technician when I leave school but I'm very shy. Can I still do the job? 99

A Clients can be a bit funny about sitting in silence while their nails are being done, and may regard you as having given poor service if you don't chat. If you're not very confident, it can feel quite hard to make conversation with a stranger, but it really is necessary, especially if you're going to be with that person for the next half hour. You would definitely need to work on your confidence – why don't you practise your manicure/nail art at school or college on people you don't know very well? You'll soon get into the swing of things.

Q 66 How can I convince a tattoo artist to take me on for an Apprenticeship? 99

A You will have to get to know some practising tattoo artists and let them see that you have the talent to do the job. You should by this stage have a portfolio prepared – this won't be composed of actual tattoos as you would not be trained or licensed to carry these out; but it should show examples of detailed accurate artwork that you have prepared yourself. You will be able to meet other tattoo artists at UK events and conventions (see websites like www.uktattoostudios.co.uk for further details). Be aware that this type of Apprenticeship does not work on the same principle as college Apprenticeship schemes.

Q 66 I know that some beauty professionals need a portfolio. What exactly is this? 99

A A portfolio is a collection of work showcasing the best pieces of work you have completed at college or work. It could include photographs, drawings or designs that show either your creative ability or your skill and it is intended to convince colleges or employers that you have the ability to work in your field. You might want to have a 'hard' copy (like a paper catalogue) so that it's portable, but it's probably better to save it on a website too – remember to include website details on your CV or college application.

> ⚡ **NEWSFLASH!**
> Victorian women drank vinegar to maintain a pale complexion.

Q 66 I asked a nail salon for an Apprenticeship and they agreed, provided I pay them £3,000. Is it worth it? 99

A This situation might happen if you live in a multicultural city – this is the way things are done in some African and Far Eastern cultures, for example. It wouldn't really be worth it, though, unless they are a very famous salon who are prepared to provide free accredited training. However, the whole idea of an Apprenticeship is that you get paid, rather than pay for it, and you will always be able to get free level 2 training until you are 19 years old, which will include some workplace experience.

Q 66 I leave school next year and I'm really interested in fashion and beauty. I want to be an image consultant: what are my first steps? 99

A A lot of young people want to be image consultants on the basis that they're creative or really enjoy fashion and beauty. It's a really good idea – but you may have to wait a few years before you can do it, building up experience and credibility as you work in another job. Fashion retail (working in a boutique) would be a good place to start, as you will gain experience of styling customers.

Q **I've just started my NVQ level 3 make-up and my tutor says I have to keep up with current trends. What does that mean?** 〞

A Of all beauty qualifications, make-up requires the most creativity. If you want to style for TV or for fashion, it is particularly important that you are aware of current trends in both fashion and culture. If you pick up *Vogue*, you will see that make-up on the catwalk changes as much as fashion, and fashion houses often have a certain theme behind their latest make-up collections. This links into cultural themes; for instance, a block-busting film like *Lord of the Rings* can influence a new look for fashion designers (this film influenced the floaty dresses/ethereal trend) and this in turn will impact on the way make-up artists style their clients. If you want to do this sort of work, you have to be the kind of person who is aware of the wider world around them.

> If you want to work in fashion and make-up, you have to be the kind of person who is aware of the wider world around them. 〞

Q 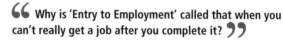 **Why is 'Entry to Employment' called that when you can't really get a job after you complete it?** 〞

A Partly because this qualification was devised some years ago when the job market was healthier than it is now, and partly because it teaches you a range of job skills that you might not otherwise have. It is preparing you for employment even if you have to do another qualification afterwards: if you haven't learned about team working, or you haven't learned to communicate properly or read and write very much, this qualification increases your chances of employment by teaching you these skills. You can think about completing an NVQ once you've finished it.

Q **Would I have to be really beautiful to work in the beauty industry?** 〞

A No, not at all. However, you should be 'well groomed' – your hair and nails should look neat and tidy and you should wear make-up.

This also applies to men, who may also choose to wear make-up – however, consider the employer first: more traditional employers might not be sympathetic to men wearing make-up. Clothing should also be neat and tidy – you will probably wear a uniform at work, but watch out for holes in your tights or scuffed shoes and be aware that customers will probably bump into you in the street and may think your 'out-of-doors' appearance reflects your beauty skills.

Q 66 **If I want to be a make-up artist, will I have to buy all my own tools?** 99

A I'm afraid you will, but you'd build them up over time, choosing the products you find more useful than others. For instance, when you start out, you can mix colours of foundations and powder products to save yourself the expense of a complete range of make-up products. And you can buy these at specialist stores which are cheaper than make-up counters. Make-up artists can be quite clever about carrying it all around, often using workmen's storage kits to carry and pack conveniently. Some beauty therapy and make-up courses will provide you with cheap starter kits, but as you progress in your career, you are likely to need a wider range of better-quality products.

> ⚡ **NEWSFLASH!**
>
> L'Oréal is the biggest cosmetics company in the world, selling €19.50 billion worth of products at the last count.

Q 66 **What would be the worst things about working in the beauty industry?** 99

A That depends on your personality – some people can't bear making small talk, for instance! Most people working in the beauty industry do seem to enjoy their work, but a customer's poor hygiene standards could be an issue for some workers. Working weekends or standing for long periods of time are often issues, but this depends on your ability to accept that this is just part of the job.

Q 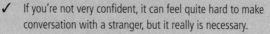 **How much holiday will I get when I'm working?**

A When you are in practice, you are entitled to a minimum of 28 days' paid holiday (including bank holidays).

> **Quick recap!**
> ✓ Don't be afraid to ask colleges or potential employers as many questions as you want: if you look as though you want the best for yourself and your future, people will respect this.
> ✓ If you're not very confident, it can feel quite hard to make conversation with a stranger, but it really is necessary.
> ✓ Take care over your personal appearance. You should look well groomed – your hair and nails should look neat and tidy and you should wear make-up.

CHAPTER 8
QUALIFICATIONS AND TRAINING

This chapter will cover the most common of the qualifications leading to jobs in the beauty industry.

THE IMPORTANCE OF GAINING GOOD QUALIFICATIONS

Skill and creativity are always going to be very important for any job in the beauty industry, but nowadays you will be also expected to have some level of qualification, as this shows at what level your skills are. Depending on the type of job you want to do, there are a number of different ways you can enter the beauty industry.

Be aware that you can achieve one level of qualification, work for a period of time and then either go back to college to gain additional qualifications, or train on the job – you don't have to wait until you have the highest qualification possible before you begin work.

> **TOP TIP!** *i*
>
> If you have any doubts at all how to choose a qualification, ask a careers adviser to help you. If you are not in education, your local council will help you find a careers adviser.

There are a vast range of qualifications available in the beauty industry and many of them will be quite expensive.

A FEW POINTS TO REMEMBER

▶ If you are above the age of 16, have already left school and are trying to choose a qualification on your own, make sure your qualification is accredited to a national awarding body. (Employers like familiarity: they need to recognise your qualifications because they need to know roughly what you've studied, the level of knowledge you have and any employability skills you would have had to show to pass the tests.)

▶ Also make sure you go to a government-funded institution: the government will not pay for courses at private colleges, but it will otherwise pay for 14- to 19-year-olds to be in education.

▶ It is likely that you will have to pay for a uniform, towels and any kit you use.

Examples of national awarding bodies for beauty qualifications are:

▶ City & Guilds
▶ Edexcel
▶ IHBC
▶ VTCT.

14–19 DIPLOMA IN HAIR AND BEAUTY

If you are still at school, take note of the 14–19 Diploma in Hair and Beauty, which has been available since September 2009. It is offered at four levels:

1. Foundation (equivalent to five GCSEs at grades D–G)
2. Higher (equivalent to seven GCSEs at grades A*–C)
3. Progression (equivalent to 2.5 A levels)
4. Advanced (equivalent to 3.5 A levels).

From this year (2011) an Extended Diploma is also available. This differs from the other levels of the Diploma by containing extra Maths, English and ICT elements as well as extra Additional and Specialist Learning. This is a level 3 qualification.

The Diploma has a vocational element but it allows you to mix a variety of subjects that interest you, without committing you to a particular career direction. Once it is completed, you can apply for work, further education, or the next part of the diploma, allowing the employer or course provider to see that you have gained a wide range of workplace and academic skills. If you have completed the Advanced Diploma, you can also consider higher education.

> ⚡ **NEWSFLASH!**
> Coco Chanel made the suntan popular in the 1920s. Before that, very white skin was the most desirable: a sign that a lady didn't have to work in the fields.

The Diploma is broken down into six parts.

1. **Principal Learning** (compulsory): an introduction to six of the best known hair and beauty industries – hairdressing, barbering, Afro-Caribbean hairdressing (e.g. corn rowing, weave), beauty therapy, spa therapy and nail services.

2. **Additional and Specialist Learning** (options you can choose): you can choose between hands-on learning (e.g. massage or complementary health) or you can choose GCSEs or A levels.

3. **Functional Skills:** you continue with English, maths and IT, but have the opportunity to see how these skills work in a practical setting.

4. **Personal, Learning and Thinking Skills:** building up your employability skills, such as teamwork, customer service skills and managing your time and workload.

5. **Work Experience:** you will get at least 10 days to help out in a workplace, perhaps helping advise customers on a make-up counter or assisting a beauty therapist in a salon. This will give you an opportunity to think about whether you like this work environment and will allow you to practise some of your employability skills.

6. **Project:** you develop and research any topic of your choice; an excellent skill to learn if you want to go to university later.

ENTRY TO EMPLOYMENT (E2E)

If you have left school with no qualifications, don't despair! There are a lot of options still available to you. E2E is available at a lot of colleges for 16- to 18-year-olds (although it is occasionally available for older students) and it's designed to teach you the skills needed for employment.

You would study beauty therapy for part of the time and you would also learn about being in the workplace. Employers don't just look for academic skills, and this course would teach you how to make the most of your time at work. For instance, you would learn about team working and how to manage your environment. You would also work on your communication and literacy skills; and you must achieve a certain level if you wish to be successful in the beauty

> **⚡ NEWSFLASH!**
> Testing cosmetics on animals was banned in the UK in 1998.

industry. Most of your work will be assessed as you do it but you would also be expected to complete basic qualifications or short courses, though these are not exam-based.

If you would like more information about E2E and vocational courses, contact your local further education college – you will be able to raise any questions or issues at their open days. Connexions also offers information on local E2E courses.

APPRENTICESHIPS

Once you have learned these essential skills (including workplace skills, such as excellent attendance and punctuality) and are already qualified to level 1 or 2, another useful way to gain entry into the beauty industry (if you feel that you are absolutely committed to the industry) is to do an Apprenticeship.

Getting acceptance onto an Apprenticeship is currently very competitive. Although they are sometimes advertised as not needing any formal qualifications, an employer will expect to see evidence that you

> ❝ Getting acceptance onto an Apprenticeship is currently very competitive. ❞

will complete the Apprenticeship and be able to pass it, and you will definitely require previous qualifications.

This means you must convince the employer that you have a record of sticking to a course, even if the going gets tough, and that you will be able to work well with their team. You will also be assessed on your English and maths and, in practice, you will generally need level 2.

You will also be expected to show basic knowledge of IT. In addition to developing your skills in a workplace setting, you will be offered two levels of college study: level 2 is the equivalent of five GCSEs (Grades A–C); and the Higher Apprenticeship (level 3) is the equivalent of A levels. Most industries increasingly demand more qualifications, which means you should aim eventually to achieve the level 3 qualification. In addition, you will be encouraged to develop your key skills further (e.g. communication and numeracy).

> 66 You must convince the employer that you have a record of sticking to a course. 99

There are two advantages of an Apprenticeship: first, it will include a very high level of workplace experience, which is important to impress future employers; second, you get paid! An apprentice gets paid no less than £2.50 per hour (although many employers pay more) and is entitled to at least 28 days' annual leave a year (including bank holidays).

The government is taking steps to link up course providers and willing employers to provide Apprenticeship 'packages', and some colleges have been following their lead. It can be quite difficult for them to find suitable employers, however, so people who wish to do an Apprenticeship should also do what they can to provide their own work placement.

Some colleges are offering Apprenticeships with employer placement 'only if available'. Be aware that without a workplace setting, you may be only training in an in-house salon: though this has value,

⚡ **NEWSFLASH!**

Henna has been used for at least 4,000 years to make beautiful patterns on the body.

employers will prefer to see that you have more 'real-world' experience, and will certainly expect to see more from an Apprenticeship.

Depending on the employer, you may be expected to take on more responsibility in the workplace than on an NVQ work placement (see 'Vocational qualifications levels 2 and 3' below). You may be asked to cover reception duties and clean and tidy treatment rooms. As a level 3 apprentice, you may expect to study modules similar to the following:

- ▶ learning about the finance and profits of a beauty business
- ▶ working according to health and safety standards
- ▶ epilation (removal of hair) in a variety of ways
- ▶ electrotherapy: using electrical beauty tools
- ▶ increasing the business's profits by promoting additional products or services, such as head and body massage treatments.

In exactly the same way as a vocational qualification, you would be assessed on the job, to see how well you communicate with customers and how well you do your treatments, but you can also expect written assignments (including case studies) and some external examinations, including separate ones for key skills (IT, English and maths).

For more information about Apprenticeships, you can also register and apply for vacancies on www.apprenticeships. org.uk. You can also contact further education colleges to see if they have Apprenticeships available – be sure to ask whether they can provide a work placement. If they can't and they expect you to organise your own, ask what kind of help they can realistically give you (for instance, can they help you sell yourself to employers and do they already have contacts with willing employers?). It's also a good idea to use local careers services, including Connexions, as they may provide useful links to employers who are willing to provide Apprenticeships.

VOCATIONAL QUALIFICATIONS LEVELS 2 AND 3 (FOR STUDENTS AGED 16 AND OVER)

If you don't want to do an Apprenticeship, but would prefer to remain in a student environment, another option is to study a variety of vocationally related qualifications at a sixth-form or further education college. Be aware that in this environment you will be studying alongside adults: this can be an advantage to those who have problems in school, as they will be more focused about their studies and provide a more serious work environment. Many of these adults will be paying considerable sums for the same course – however, if you begin your course aged 16–18, you will receive government funding for all of your course fees.

Qualifications of this type include BTEC, NVQ and City & Guilds Diplomas and are available for specific jobs (mentioned in Chapter 3). These qualifications last between one and two years. The most basic qualification in this range is at level 1, which is equivalent to five GCSEs at Grade D–G.

You might expect to study the following modules on a level 1 beauty therapy course:

▶ assisting with manicures
▶ assisting with skincare and facials
▶ working on the salon reception, helping to answer general queries and greet clients
▶ health and safety
▶ communication and IT.

It is preferable to study at levels 2 and 3 as you are more likely to gain employment at these levels. You will also see HNDs advertised – these are level 4.

As an example of a level 2 course, if you wish to study nail technology, you might expect to study:

▶ health and safety (e.g. disposing of waste)
▶ a background to working in the nail industry
▶ advising clients on nail treatments and helping them choose designs
▶ providing manicure and pedicure treatments
▶ providing nail art services
▶ working on reception
▶ promoting sales in a salon
▶ stock-taking: assessing and re-ordering stock.

A level 2 or 3 beauty therapy course would still be acting as an introduction to a number of roles in the beauty industry. You might expect to study:

▶ health and safety
▶ eyelash and eyebrow treatments
▶ working on reception
▶ assessing and improving facial skin condition
▶ marketing additional products or services
▶ manicures
▶ pedicures
▶ removing hair using waxing techniques.

You might also study modules on hair styling and basic make-up.

There are also a large variety of level 2 and 3 courses available for body massage therapy, some of which, like the City & Guilds level 3 Diploma in Anatomy, Physiology and Pathology, will require more scientific knowledge than others. You may choose to specialise in aromatherapy, Swedish massage or many other types on offer, or you may wish to combine courses, but these courses do tend to be non-accredited (meaning you won't get funding), so you may want to wait until you're working before you either get on-the-job training or you are in a position to pay for it yourself.

⚡ NEWSFLASH!

Men are more likely to have medical aesthetic treatments in London, Cardiff and Swindon than anywhere else in the UK.

IF YOU WANT TO WORK ABROAD . . .

If you know that you want to work abroad eventually, it may be worth your while considering an ITEC course in your subject. ITEC courses are recognised in 33 countries and are available at levels 2 and 3 and in a wide range of subjects, including beauty, nail technology and ear piercing.

There is also a BTEC Retail Beauty Consultancy Diploma (level 2) available at the London College of Beauty Therapy, which could give you the edge over the competition if you were committed to a career in beauty consultancy. You would expect to study a combination of courses, including customer service, how to make sales, how to build good customer relationships, health and safety, and security. You will also be taught the basics of nail care, perfumery, skincare and make-up application.

> 66 Employers still prize good presentation, good product knowledge, sales skills and a friendly approach over a formal qualification. 99

However, this qualification is not currently a necessity: employers still prize good presentation, good product knowledge, sales skills and a friendly approach over a formal qualification.

If you wish to study make-up to work in salons or on a catwalk or in magazines, you may find it useful to study at a specialist college or to consider a level 2 BTEC or NVQ in make-up level 2 or 3. You could additionally follow specialist make-up modules as part of a beauty therapy qualification, and you should make sure this option is available to you before enrolling on your course.

The qualification may help you find work in salons, but in itself it won't find you work in fashion – however, it will improve your knowledge of application and provide you with important practical skills. Level 3 qualifications that introduce you to theatrical and media make-up may provide useful employer links – some employers approach colleges to ask students to help with a particular production.

This is useful for the employer if they are on a tight budget and want to save money on labour costs; and it is useful to the student in terms of gaining very valuable work experience, building a portfolio and gaining opportunities to network for future employment opportunities.

If working as a salon receptionist appeals to you, you may not need any qualifications, though you will have to demonstrate intermediate IT skills and an interest in the beauty industry. Some salon receptionists have taken an NVQ beauty therapy level 1.

> 66 If you negotiate well with your employer and clients, they can provide the workplace setting within which you can be assessed. 99

It's a good idea to show employers that you have English and maths GCSEs and you might consider studying for business administration level 2. Once you are in this job, you may consider new or further beauty qualifications – if you negotiate well with your employer and clients, they can provide the workplace setting within which you can be assessed.

You could also consider an Access to Beauty course which is designed to get you through to higher education and therefore has a higher academic content than level 3 vocational qualifications. You will still learn a variety of practical beauty techniques but you will also be learning about how to learn in higher education (study skills).

The advantage is that a university may look upon an Access course more favourably than an NVQ level 3, as it is specifically geared towards getting you into university, but the disadvantage is that it will be harder to gain employment with it as a stand-alone qualification. There is a much higher written content in an Access course than a vocational course.

TOP TIP!

You should keep in mind, when choosing a course, that the beauty industry is one that strongly prefers practical experience to academic ability, but do use every opportunity to gain qualifications while you are working.

CIBTAC/CIDESCO

If you are 18 years old or above and you have completed level 3 qualifications, you might consider completing the internationally recognised CIBTAC (Confederation of International Beauty Therapy and Cosmetology) and CIDESCO (Comité International d'Esthétique et de Cosmétologie) diplomas – despite the French name, they are widely available at UK colleges. No previous beauty experience is required for these courses, so they may be a useful option if you have reached level 3 in unrelated subjects, but now feel you want to enter the beauty industry.

These are very comprehensive and prestigious programmes of salon techniques at the same level as Foundation degrees, but concentrating on the practical side (though you will also have to write a 4,000-word thesis). Both CIBTAC and CIDESCO are offered by private colleges and you will not be able to access public funding to support your tuition fees – 2011/12 fees ranged from £7,250 to £9,700 for the year's course at UK colleges.

HIGHER EDUCATION

Nowadays, vocational qualifications can lead to higher education and there are a number of beauty therapy courses available that are designed for those who are now managing their own salons, or who would like to do so. As part of these courses, you will continue developing your salon techniques but you will also learn the practicalities of running a business, legal matters relevant to the beauty industry and managing staff.

> ## ⚡ NEWSFLASH!
> Beauty therapists can even find employment in the armed forces or the prison service.

Courses include Foundation degrees or HNDs in beauty therapy, spa management and make-up design, and some universities may ask for traditional GCSE and A level passes rather than vocational beauty qualifications. In practice, however, if you have considerable knowledge and experience of the beauty industry, entry may be more flexible.

TEACHING

Once you have gained experience in the industry, you might want to consider teaching. You don't have to train in the same way as a school teacher but you will have to be qualified to level 3 in your own subject and may then choose to do an A1 Assessor Award or take a level 3 and 4 certificate or level 5 Diploma in Teaching in the Lifelong Learning Sector.

So, if you wanted to become an NVQ beauty therapy teacher, you would have level 3 qualifications in beauty therapy, and work experience, and you would train as an assessor while you were working as a beauty therapist (you would need to provide your workplace as a work placement from which you would be assessed).

Additionally, you could choose to complete the 7303 (PTLLS – Preparing to Teach in the Lifelong Learning Sector), a 10-week introduction to teaching course. This could be followed by the 7304 (CTLLS – Certificate to Teach in the Lifelong Learning Sector), a six-month course which requires you to do 30 hours of teaching and observing in a placement (you need a mentor in this placement).

ADDITIONAL QUALIFICATIONS

Most work for image consultants is found through networking, building up a reputation and advertising and most image consultants have done this in the fashion industry. Image consultants rarely look for specific qualifications, though some private personal styling companies do offer them, and you might consider them once you've built up good customer service experience and you're able to pay for them (you won't get government funding).

⚡ **NEWSFLASH!**

The red dye in lipstick comes from carminic acid – which is produced from dried insects.

Some specialist colleges such as St Martin's College or the London School of Fashion may offer accredited qualifications which are relevant, though focused on the fashion rather than the beauty industry. You might consider a year's study at a fashion college, as a way of getting onto

ACCESS TO THE BEAUTY INDUSTRY

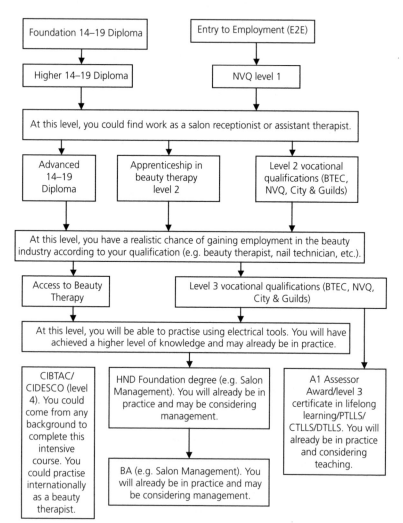

Foundation 14–19 Diploma

Entry to Employment (E2E)

Higher 14–19 Diploma

NVQ level 1

At this level, you could find work as a salon receptionist or assistant therapist.

Advanced 14–19 Diploma

Apprenticeship in beauty therapy level 2

Level 2 vocational qualifications (BTEC, NVQ, City & Guilds)

At this level, you have a realistic chance of gaining employment in the beauty industry according to your qualification (e.g. beauty therapist, nail technician, etc.).

Access to Beauty Therapy

Level 3 vocational qualifications (BTEC, NVQ, City & Guilds)

At this level, you will be able to practise using electrical tools. You will have achieved a higher level of knowledge and may already be in practice.

CIBTAC/ CIDESCO (level 4). You could come from any background to complete this intensive course. You could practise internationally as a beauty therapist.

HND Foundation degree (e.g. Salon Management). You will already be in practice and may be considering management.

A1 Assessor Award/level 3 certificate in lifelong learning/PTLLS/ CTLLS/DTLLS. You will already be in practice and considering teaching.

BA (e.g. Salon Management). You will already be in practice and may be considering management.

a fashion degree – and you could then top up your skills by completing short courses in make-up or nail technology.

Beauty journalists do not necessarily need any beauty qualifications, though the knowledge gained from these would be very useful. Many journalists have degrees and some have completed courses in journalism such as those offered by the National Council for the Training of Journalists (NCTJ).

The Access to the Beauty Industry chart on the previous page is an overview of how qualifications in the beauty industry work. The UK qualification system changes rapidly and repeatedly and you should bear in mind two important points.

1. New qualifications can initially be viewed with suspicion by HE/FE providers, who may be unsure of what students have attained. At the time of writing not all educational providers have categorically stated that they will accept the new 14–19 Diplomas or the Advanced Apprenticeship as a basis for higher education.

2. Colleges will provide their own assessments at every stage and may be significantly more flexible than the chart indicates.

Quick recap!
✓ You can achieve one level of qualification, work for a period of time and then go back to college to gain additional qualifications.
✓ There are two advantages to an Apprenticeship: first, there will be a very high level of workplace experience, which is important to impress future employers; second, you get paid.
✓ Skill and creativity are very important for any job in the beauty industry.

CHAPTER 9
REAL LIVES 3

DAVE O'SULLIVAN: TATTOO ARTIST

Dave has been a tattoo artist for 15 years and has recently opened his own studio in south London.

'I've always loved drawing,' says Dave. 'I'm actually dyslexic so when I was at school, I struggled with my classes a bit – but I always had a real talent for drawing accurately. You don't have to be a great artist to be a tattooist but it's important to be accurate.'

> 66 You don't have to be a great artist to be a tattooist but it's important to be accurate. 99

Dave already knew a number of tattoo artists by the time he left school, so he knew a bit about how the work was performed and about the work environment. He tried to get an Apprenticeship but found this difficult, as artists don't always like to share their expertise. Instead, he concentrated on attending conventions to build up his product knowledge (and knowledge of where to buy products) and he also began to practise on himself.

'It's actually necessary for you to start out on yourself anyway,' he points out, 'because you'll have to understand what it actually feels like to have a tattoo done. It is painful and you have to know how you react to it, because if you have a customer who reacts unexpectedly, it'll spoil your design.' The process should be supervised by an experienced tattooist, however, as it could be quite dangerous if you did it on your own.

Dave was able to show his own designs at the conventions and he managed to gain a reputation this way. 'We've come a long way from just tattooing "Mum and Dad" on people: there are some really good artists out there: highly experimental; and more and more people are doing it so there's a greater pool of ideas. More women are getting involved now.'

> 66 You should be careful to work for a licensed studio – they're strict about following heath and safety procedures. 99

Because he gained a good reputation, he found work with a studio licensed by the local health authority, and he was then free to practise on customers. 'You should be careful to work for a licensed studio – they're strict about following heath and safety procedures, like disposing of waste contaminated by blood. You can also buy better products, like colours, from specialist companies who will only sell to registered studios.'

Dave's earnings vary: his work tends to be seasonal and more customers will want tattoos in the summer months

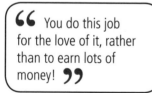

> 66 You do this job for the love of it, rather than to earn lots of money! 99

when they can show them off. The winter months can leave him out of pocket, especially as he has just opened a new business, so it's really important that he enjoys the job itself – he loves creating new designs. 'It takes about three or four years to develop a studio like this – I'll spread the word with flyers, on the internet and largely through word of mouth, but this month, my earnings average out at about £1 per hour. Of course, it's not always like that, but you can see why you do this job for the love of it, rather than to earn lots of money!'

And Dave really does love his job: 'Where else would I get to show my artwork? I wouldn't be the type of person to have paintings in art galleries, so this is how I create art. There's nothing to beat the satisfaction of seeing a piece of living artwork actually walking around – and I've actually created that. I like to see the pride my clients have in actually getting through the procedure, as well, because it can be quite an ordeal for them sometimes!'

> 66 There's nothing to beat the satisfaction of seeing a piece of living artwork actually walking around. 99

It doesn't always go well, though. Even though Dave is very quick with his tattoos, some clients still move too much because of the pain, and this causes Dave to make mistakes. 'You definitely need good customer service skills at all times, but you particularly need diplomacy in this situation because if they don't keep still, you're going to have to get rid of them. What you can't afford is for bad artwork to be walking around – it just spoils your reputation and your reputation is everything in this game.'

TOP TIP! *i*

Attend as many conventions as possible – that way you build up contacts, ideas and new materials and can make informed decisions about whether you want to do tattooing for a living.

If you're thinking of becoming a tattoo artist, Dave's advice would be to 'have confidence in your own ability. You have to work speedily, because that means greater accuracy, so you just have to do it and not spend the time worrying.'

CHAPTER 10
THE LAST WORD

After having read this book, you should have a better idea of whether the beauty industry is suited to you. The next section will provide you with further information, but before you continue your research, ask yourself some basic questions.

Do you already have enthusiasm for reading beauty product news?	☐ Yes	☐ No
Are you prepared to take beauty qualifications, practising pedicures and facials for long periods until they're perfect?	☐ Yes	☐ No
Are you prepared to continually learn new beauty techniques and *keep* taking new qualifications, even when you've got a job?	☐ Yes	☐ No
Do you enjoy working with other people who are interested in beauty?	☐ Yes	☐ No
Do you enjoy keeping yourself well presented and taking trouble every morning with your own appearance?	☐ Yes	☐ No
Are you comfortable starting and maintaining conversations with strangers?	☐ Yes	☐ No

Are you a tactful and diplomatic sort of person?	☐ Yes ☐ No
Are you patient enough to concentrate and get every last detail right when creating a very complicated design for nails?	☐ Yes ☐ No

If you answered 'Yes' to all these questions, congratulations! You've chosen the right career. If you've answered 'No' to any of these questions, a career as a beauty professional may not be for you: however, there are still plenty of other jobs involving beauty/personal appearance that may suit you better – retail or fashion, for example. Above all, examine your reasons for choosing a career in beauty and concentrate on the things you like. For example, if you love make-up or beauty products, but feel that you lack the creativity to be a make-up artist, you could consider a job in business-to-business cosmetics sales (e.g. selling cosmetics to salons). If you like the idea of helping people on a one-to-one basis, for instance, but you're not really that interested in beauty products, there are a whole range of jobs in customer service, including retail, that might suit you better. If it's the beauty environment you like, for instance you really want to work on a cruise ship or in a salon, you could consider administration or a range of logistical jobs, such as catering, that would take place in the same environment. The key is to be honest with yourself and identify what really motivates you.

Hopefully this book has already answered many of your questions and concerns. If not, try and do a bit of research from the resources listed in the next chapter, or ask your careers adviser for additional information.

CHAPTER 11
FURTHER INFORMATION

There is a formidable amount of information on the beauty industry available to you on the internet and in the media. Below are listed some of the most reliable UK sources, which should be able to answer any questions you have about the industry.

OVERVIEW OF THE BEAUTY INDUSTRY

Cruisemates
www.cruisemates.com

If you're wondering what it's like to work on a cruise ship, take a look at this website, which is written by experienced crew. Good information on rankings, working terms and conditions and what you can expect from life on board.

Habia (Hairdressing and Beauty Industry Authority)
Tel: 0845 230 6080
www.habia.org

Habia sets standards for accredited beauty-related
qualifications and regulates the industry's codes of practice.
It can provide basic information on qualifications, including
Apprenticeships and the new Diploma in Hair and Beauty,
and provides information on forthcoming beauty events.

Jobs 4 U
www.connexions-direct.com/jobs4u/index.cfm

This is a Connexions website which breaks down job
profiles in the same way as the Careers Advice Service
[see above] and provides supplementary information.

Next Step Careers Advice Service
www.nextstep.direct.gov.uk

Offers career profiles on a variety of beauty jobs, including
a skills section and information on where to find vacancies
(useful if you are coming to the end of your course). It also
provides advice on potential salaries, though this reflects
wages outside London.

QUALIFICATIONS

Visit your local colleges' websites for information on
E2E courses and NVQs. These will provide preliminary
information on what to expect from each course and
information on what qualifications you need to have
in order to apply. More in-depth information on course
modules should be available at open days.

Apprenticeships
www.apprenticeships.org.uk

You can register on the website to search for vacancies in your area. This website has a thorough FAQ section for potential students and their parents.

City & Guilds
Tel: 020 7294 2800
www.cityandguilds.com

For information and answers to questions on vocational qualifications (including Apprenticeships) in beauty therapy.

London College of Beauty Therapy
Tel: 020 7208 1300/1301
www.lcbt.co.uk

Information on workplace learning courses, including Diploma in Beauty Retail Consultancy level 2.

London College of Fashion
Tel: 020 7514 7400
www.fashion.arts.ac.uk

Provides information on higher education and short courses in beauty therapy, make-up and cosmetic science. Visit the website or phone to book onto one of their open days.

UCAS
www.ucas.ac.uk

UCAS can provide information on where to study beauty-related degrees, when to apply for them and what qualifications you already need in place before you apply.

INDUSTRY NEWS

Magazines

Keep your eye on magazines such as *Vogue* for the latest news on beauty and cosmetic products. Although many of these products may be too expensive to buy and test, these publications often include useful information on what ingredients have been used and which are currently popular. They also contain information about what beauty treatments are currently the most popular. You can buy cheaper publications than *Vogue* – but they won't have the same quality of information.

YouTube

Don't miss a visit to YouTube – an enormous variety of people provide advice on beauty and make-up. You'll have to wade through, sifting the good from the bad, but the good is very, very good indeed! You will find that communities share information on the industry's latest products, and many independently review them – handy if you don't want to test everything on the market. You might even make some useful contacts!

Creative Nail Design
www.cnd.com

If nail art and technology is your passion, visit this website and take a look at the 'Look Book' and Style Gallery for up-to-date inspiration, including their leopard-print nail designs.